THE

OBESITY CODE

AMAZING FORMULAR FOR WEIGHT LOSS

WITHOUT STRESS

JASON BRYSON PETERSON

INTRODUCTION

The term obesity portrays an individual who's exceptionally overweight, with a great deal of muscle to fat ratio.

It's a typical issue in the UK that is evaluated to influence around 1 in each 4 grown-ups and around 1 in each 5 kids matured 10 to 11.

The most generally utilized strategy to check in case you're a solid weight is weight list (BMI).

BMI is a proportion of whether you're a solid load for your tallness. You can utilize the BMI solid weight number cruncher to work out your score. It's imperative to find a way to handle corpulence in light of the fact that, just as causing evident physical transforms, it can prompt various genuine and conceivably perilous conditions. Weight is by and large brought about by expending more calories, especially those in greasy and sugary nourishments, than you consume physical movement. The overabundance vitality is put away by the body as fat. The most ideal approach to treat obesity is to eat a solid diminished calorie diet and exercise routinely. at times, weight reduction medical procedure might be prescribed.

TABLE OF CONTENTS

CHAPTER ONE 1

WHAT IS OBESITY? 1

CAUSES 2

CHAPTER TWO 19

SYMPTOMS OF OBESITY 19

THE OBESITY EPIDEMIC 22

CHAPTER THREE 25

CHILDHOOD OBESITY 25

HEALTH EFFECTS OF OBESITY 30

CHAPTER FOUR 34

TREATMENT OF OBESITY 34

OBESE PERSONS ARE PRESCRIBED TO: 37

OBESITY AND EXERCISE 42

CHAPTER ONE

WHAT IS OBESITY?

Obesity, likewise called rotundity or corpulence, unreasonable amassing of muscle versus fat, as a rule brought about by the utilization of a greater number of calories than the body can utilize. The abundance calories are then put away as fat, or fat tissue. Overweight, if moderate, isn't really heftiness, especially in strong or huge boned people.

Obesity is an ailment that happens when an individual conveys overabundance weight or muscle to fat ratio that may influence their wellbeing. A specialist will for the most part propose that an individual has corpulence on the off chance that they have a high body mass index.

Body Mass Index (BMI) is an apparatus that specialists use to survey if an individual is at a suitable load for their age, sex, and stature. The estimation joins tallness and weight.

A BMI somewhere in the range of 25 and 29.9 shows that an individual is conveying overabundance weight. A BMI of 30 or over recommends that an individual may have weight.

CAUSES

Different factors, for example, the proportion of waist to-hip size (WHR), waist-to-height-ratio (WtHR), and the sum and dissemination of fat on the body likewise assume a job in deciding how sound an individual's weight and body shape are.

In the event that an individual has stoutness and abundance weight, this can expand their danger of building up various wellbeing conditions, including metabolic disorder, joint inflammation, and a few kinds of disease.

Metabolic disorder includes a gathering of issues, for example, hypertension, type 2 diabetes, and cardiovascular illness.

Keeping up a sound weight or losing through diet and exercise is one approach to avoid or decrease corpulence. At times, an individual may require medical procedure.

Presently read on to discover why obesity occurs.

1) CONSUMING TOO MUCH CALORIES

At the point when an individual expends a bigger number of calories than they use as vitality, their body will store the additional calories as fat. This can prompt abundance weight and corpulence.

Additionally, a few sorts of nourishments are bound to prompt weight gain, particularly those that are high in fats and sugars.

Nourishments that will in general increment the danger of weight addition include:

- Fast foods

- seared nourishments, for example, French fries
- greasy and prepared meats
- numerous dairy items
- foods with included sugar, for example, heated products, instant breakfast grains, and treats
- foods containing concealed sugars, for example, ketchup and numerous other canned and bundled nourishment things
- improved juices, soft drinks, and mixed drinks
- prepared, high-carb nourishments, for example, bread and bagels

Some prepared nourishment items contain high-fructose corn syrup as a sugar, including appetizing things, for example, ketchup.

Eating a lot of these nourishments and doing too little exercise can bring about weight addition and stoutness.

An individual who devours an eating regimen that comprises for the most part of natural products, vegetables, entire grains, and water is still in danger of putting on overabundance weight on the off chance that they gorge, or if hereditary factors, for instance, increment their hazard.

Be that as it may, they are bound to appreciate a differed eating regimen while keeping up a solid weight. Crisp nourishments and entire grains contain fiber, which makes an individual vibe full for more and supports solid assimilation.

2) LEADING A SEDENTARY LIFESTYLE

Numerous individuals lead a substantially more inactive way of life than their folks and grandparents.

Instances of stationary propensities include:

working in an office as opposed to doing physical work

messing around on a PC as opposed to doing physical exercises outside

going to places via vehicle as opposed to strolling or cycling

The less an individual moves around, the less calories they consume.

Likewise, physical action influences how an individual's hormones work, and hormones affect how the body forms nourishment.

A few studies have indicated that physical action can keep insulin levels stable and that flimsy insulin levels may prompt weight gain.

Analysts who distributed a review Trusted Source in BMJ Open Sport and Exercise Medicine in 2017 noticed that, while the structures of certain investigations make it difficult to make definite inferences, "A way of life consolidating standard [physical activity] has been recognized as a key factor for keeping up and improving numerous parts of wellbeing, including insulin affectability."

Physical action need not be preparing in the recreation center. Physical work, strolling or cycling, climbing stairs, and family unit assignments all contribute.

Nonetheless, the sort and force of action may influence how much it benefits the body in the short-and long haul.

3) NOT SLEEPING ENOUGH

Research has recommended that missing rest builds the danger of putting on weight and creating corpulence.

Scientists checked on proof for more than 28,000 youngsters and 15,000 grown-ups in the United Kingdom from 1977 to 2012. In 2012, they presumed that lack of sleep essentially expanded stoutness chance in the two grown-ups and youngsters.

The progressions influenced youngsters as youthful as 5 years old.

The group recommended that lack of sleep may prompt corpulence since it can prompt hormonal changes that expansion the hunger.

At the point when an individual doesn't rest enough, their body produces ghrelin, a hormone that animates craving. Simultaneously, an absence of rest likewise brings about a lower generation of leptin, a hormone that smothers the hunger.

4) ENDOCRINE DISRUPTORS

A group from the University of Barcelona distributed a study Trusted Source in the World Journal of Gastroenterology that gives pieces of information with respect to how fluid fructose — a kind of sugar — in drinks may change lipid vitality digestion and lead to greasy liver and metabolic disorder.

Highlights of metabolic disorder incorporate diabetes, cardiovascular malady, and hypertension. Individuals with stoutness are bound to have metabolic disorder.

Subsequent to encouraging rodents a 10-percent fructose answer for 14 days, the researchers noticed that their digestion was beginning to change.

Researchers accept there is a connection between high utilization of fructose and weight and metabolic disorder. Specialists have raised worries about the utilization of high-fructose corn syrup to improve drinks and other nourishment items.

Creature studies have discovered that when weight happens because of fructose utilization, there is likewise a nearby connection with type 2 diabetes.

In 2018, specialists distributed the consequences of examinations including youthful rodents. They, too experienced metabolic changes, oxidative pressure, and aggravation in the wake of devouring fructose syrup.

The analysts note that "expanded fructose admission might be a significant indicator of metabolic hazard in youngsters."

They call for changes in the eating regimens of youngsters to forestall these issues.

5) MEDICATIONS AND WEIGHT GAIN

A few drugs can likewise prompt weight gain.

Aftereffects of an audit and meta-analysisTrusted Source distributed in The Journal of Clinical Endocrinology and Metabolism in 2015 found that a few medications made individuals put on weight over a time of months.

atypical antipsychotics, particularly olanzapine, quetiapine, and risperidone

Anticonvulsants and mind-set stabilizers, and explicitly gabapentin

hypoglycemic meds, for example, tolbutamide

glucocorticoids used to treat rheumatoid joint inflammation

A few antidepressants

Notwithstanding, a few meds may prompt weight reduction. Any individual who is beginning another medicine and is worried about their weight ought to ask their PCP whether the medication is probably going to have any impact on weight.

6) IS OBESITY SELF-PERPETUATING?

The more drawn out an individual is overweight, the harder it might be for them to get more fit.

Discoveries of a mouse study Trusted Source, distributed in the diary Nature Communications in 2015, proposed that the more fat an individual conveys, the more outlandish the body is to copy fat, in light of a protein, or quality, known as sLR11.

It appears that the more fat an individual has, the more sLR11 their body will deliver. The protein obstructs the body's capacity to consume fat, making it harder to shed the additional weight.

7) OBESITY GENE

A defective quality called the fat-mass and heftiness related quality (FTO) is liable for certain instances of corpulence.

A study distributed in 2013 points to a connection between this quality and:

Weight

Practices that lead to weight

A higher nourishment admission

An inclination for unhealthy nourishments

A debilitated capacity to feel full, known as satiety

The hormone ghrelin assumes a vital job in eating conduct. Ghrelin additionally affects Trusted Source the arrival of development hormones and how the body collects fat, among different capacities.

The action of the FTO quality may affect an individual's odds of having weight since it influences the measures of ghrelin an individual has.

In a study Trusted Source including 250 individuals with dietary issues, distributed in Plos One of every

2017, specialists proposed that parts of FTO may likewise assume a job in conditions, for example, gorging and enthusiastic eating.

Numerous components assume a job in the advancement of stoutness. Hereditary characteristics can build the hazard in certain individuals.

A stimulating eating routine that contains a lot of new nourishment, together with normal work out, will decrease the danger of weight in the vast majority.

Be that as it may, those that have a hereditary inclination may think that its harder to keep up a solid weigh

CHAPTER TWO

SYMPTOMS OF OBESITY

Being somewhat overweight may not cause numerous observable issues. Notwithstanding, when you are conveying a couple of additional kilograms, you may create indications that influence your day by day life.

Medical issues

Obesity can make day medical issues, for example,

windedness

expanded perspiring

wheezing

failure to adapt to abrupt physical action

feeling tired each day

back and joint pains

low certainty and confidence

feeling secluded

Corpulence can likewise cause transforms you may not see, however that can truly hurt your wellbeing, for example, (hypertension) and elevated cholesterol levels (greasy stores hindering your conduits). The two conditions essentially increment your danger of building up a cardiovascular sickness, for example,

coronary illness, which may prompt a cardiovascular failure

stroke, which can cause noteworthy inability and can be lethal

Another long haul issue that can influence hefty individuals is type 2 diabetes. It is assessed that simply under portion of all instances of diabetes are connected to corpulence. The primary indications of diabetes are:

feeling parched

setting off to the can a ton, particularly around evening time

outrageous tiredness

Obesity can add to numerous other ceaseless conditions, including a few malignancies, some asthma, back issues, incessant kidney malady, dementia, gallbladder ailment, gout, and osteoarthritis. Being overweight or hefty is additionally connected with passing on rashly.

Mental issues

Notwithstanding the everyday medical issues, numerous individuals may likewise encounter mental issues.

These can influence associations with relatives and companions and may prompt sorrow.

THE OBESITY EPIDEMIC

Body weight is affected by the association of numerous elements. There is solid proof of hereditary inclination to fat amassing, and corpulence will in general run in families. Be that as it may, the ascent in corpulence in populaces worldwide since the 1980s has outpaced the rate at which hereditary changes are regularly joined into populaces on a huge scale. Moreover, developing quantities of people in parts of the reality where corpulence was once uncommon have additionally put on unnecessary weight. As per the World Health Organization (WHO), which considered worldwide weight a scourge, in 2016 more than 1.9 billion grown-ups (age 18 or more seasoned) worldwide were overweight and 650 million, speaking to 13 percent of the world's grown-up populace, were hefty.

The commonness of overweight and weight fluctuated crosswise over nations, crosswise over towns and urban areas inside nations, and crosswise over populaces of people. In China and Japan, for example, the stoutness rate for people was around 5 percent, yet in certain urban communities in China it had move to almost 20 percent. In 2005 it was discovered that in excess of 70 percent of Mexican ladies were stout. WHO overview information discharged in 2010 uncovered that the greater part of the individuals living in nations in the Pacific Islands locale were overweight, with somewhere in the range of 80 percent of ladies in American Samoa saw as stout.

CHAPTER THREE

CHILDHOOD OBESITY

Childhood obesity has become a significant problem in many countries. Overweight children often face stigma and suffer from emotional, psychological, and social problems. Obesity can negatively impact a child's education and future socioeconomic status. In 2004 an estimated nine million American children over age six, including teenagers, were overweight, or obese (the terms were typically used interchangeably in describing excess fatness in children). Moreover, in the 1980s and 1990s the prevalence of obesity had more than doubled among children age 2 to 5 (from 5 percent to 10 percent) and age 6 to 11 (from

6 percent to 15 percent). By 2015, 20 percent of children age 6 to 19 were obese in the United States. Further estimates in some rural areas of the country indicated that more than 30 percent of school-age children suffered from obesity. Similar increases were seen in other parts of the world. In the United Kingdom, for example, the prevalence of obesity among children age 2 to 10 had increased from 10 percent in 1995 to 14 percent in 2003, and data from a study conducted there in 2007 indicated that 23 percent of children age 4 to 5 and 32 percent of children age 10 to 11 were overweight or obese. By 2016, WHO data indicated, worldwide some 41

million children age 5 or under were overweight or obese.

In 2005 the American Academy of Pediatrics called obesity "the pediatric epidemic of the new millennium." Overweight and obese children were increasingly diagnosed with high blood pressure, elevated cholesterol, and type II diabetes mellitus—conditions once seen almost exclusively in adults. In addition, overweight children experience broken bones and problems with joints more often than normal-weight children. The long-term consequences of obesity in young people are of great concern to pediatricians and public health experts because obese children are at high risk of becoming obese adults. Experts on longevity have concluded that today's American youth might "live less healthy and possibly even shorter lives than their parents" if the rising prevalence of obesity is left unchecked.

Curbing the rise in childhood obesity was the aim of the Alliance for a Healthier Generation, a partnership formed in 2005 by the American Heart Association, former U.S. president Bill Clinton, and the children's television network Nickelodeon. The alliance intended to reach kids through a vigorous public-awareness campaign. Similar projects followed, including American first lady Michelle Obama's Let's Move! program, launched in 2010, and campaigns against overweight and obesity were made in other countries as well.

Efforts were also under way to develop more-effective childhood obesity-prevention strategies, including the development of methods capable of predicting infants' risk of later becoming overweight or obese. One such tool reported in 2012 was found to successfully predict newborn obesity risk by taking into account newborn weight, maternal and paternal BMI, the number of members in the newborn's household, maternal occupational status, and maternal smoking during pregnancy.

HEALTH EFFECTS OF OBESITY
Stoutness might be bothersome from a tasteful sense, particularly in parts of the existence where slimness is the prominent inclination, however it is likewise a genuine restorative issue. For the most part, corpulent people have a shorter future; they endure prior, all the more frequently, and all the more seriously from an enormous number of ailments than do their ordinary weight partners. For instance, individuals who are stout are additionally much of the time influenced by diabetes; truth be told, around the world, about 90 percent of type II diabetes cases are brought about by overabundance weight. Corpulence is additionally a critical reason for malignancy; by

2018, overweight and stoutness were liable for around 1 in each 25 tumors analyzed around the world. In the United States, specialists found that the frequency of heftiness related disease was expanding among moderately youthful grown-ups matured 25 to 49.

The relationship among weight and the decay of cardiovascular wellbeing, which shows in conditions, for example, diabetes and hypertension (unusually hypertension), places fat people in danger for quickened psychological decrease as they age. Examinations of cerebrum size in people with long haul corpulence uncovered that expanded muscle to fat ratio is related with the decay (squandering ceaselessly) of mind tissue, especially in the transient and frontal flaps of the cerebrum. Truth be told, both overweight and corpulence, and along these lines a BMI of 25 or higher, are related with decreases in mind size, which builds the danger of dementia, the most widely recognized type of which is Alzheimer infection.

Obese ladies are regularly influenced by fruitlessness, taking more time to imagine than ordinary weight ladies, and fat ladies who become pregnant are at an expanded danger of unsuccessful labor. Men who are stout are additionally at expanded danger of richness issues, since abundance muscle versus fat is related with diminished testosterone levels. By and large, comparative with ordinary weight people, fat people are bound to kick the bucket rashly of degenerative maladies of the heart, corridors, and kidneys, and they have an expanded danger of creating malignancy. Hefty people additionally have an expanded danger of death from mishaps and establish poor careful dangers. Psychological wellness is influenced; conduct results of a large appearance, running from modesty and withdrawal to excessively strong self-attestation, might be established in depressions and psychoses.

CHAPTER FOUR

TREATMENT OF OBESITY

The treatment of heftiness has two fundamental destinations: evacuation of the causative components, which might be troublesome if the causes are of enthusiastic or mental source, and expulsion of surplus fat by lessening nourishment admission. Come back to typical body weight by decreasing calorie admission is best done under restorative supervision. Dietary crazes and lessening consumes less calories that produce snappy results without exertion are of farfetched viability in diminishing body weight and holding it down, and most are really pernicious to wellbeing. (See eating fewer carbs.) Weight misfortune is best accomplished through expanded physical action and essential dietary changes, for example, bringing down all out calorie admission by substituting foods grown from the ground for refined sugars.

A few medications are affirmed for the treatment of corpulence. Two of them are Belviq (lorcaserin hydrochloride) and Qsymia (phentermine and topiramate). Belviq diminishes large people's longings for sugar rich nourishments by animating the arrival of serotonin, which typically is activated via starch admission. Qsymia use the weight reduction reactions of topiramate, an antiepileptic tranquilize, and the stimulant properties of phentermine, a current momentary treatment for heftiness.

Phentermine recently had been a piece of fen-phen (fenfluramine-phentermine), an antiobesity mix that was expelled from the U.S. advertise in 1997 in light of the high hazard for heart valve harm related with fenfluramine.

OBESITY AND DIET

A great many people should decrease their day by day kilojoule admission so as to get more fit. This implies eating and drinking less and settling on more advantageous nourishment decisions. One approach to do this is to swap unfortunate and high vitality nourishment decisions, for example, inexpensive food, prepared nourishment and sugary drinks (counting liquor) for more beneficial decisions.

OBESE PERSONS ARE PRESCRIBED TO:

appreciate a wide assortment of nutritious nourishments from these five gatherings consistently:

vegetables, including various sorts and hues, and vegetables/beans

natural product

grain (oat) nourishments, for the most part wholegrain as well as high oat fiber assortments, for example, bread, oats, rice, pasta, noodles, polenta, couscous, oats, quinoa and grain.

lean meats and poultry, fish, eggs, tofu, nuts and seeds, and vegetables/beans (the last in two nutritional categories as they are wealthy in protein and starches)

milk, yogurt, cheddar as well as their other options, generally diminished fat (decreased fat milks are not reasonable for youngsters under 2 years)

drink a lot of water

limit admission of nourishments containing soaked fat, included salt, included sugars and liquor

A few cafés, bistros and cheap food outlets give kilojoules data per divide, however giving this data isn't necessary. Be cautious - a few nourishments can rapidly take you over the breaking point, for example, burgers and seared chicken.

Maintain a strategic distance from prevailing fashion eats less carbs

Maintain a strategic distance from prevailing fashion consumes less calories that suggest dangerous practices, for example, extraordinary fasting or removing whole nutrition types, for example, meat, fish, wheat or dairy items.

These are not feasible, can make you feel sick, and may cause terrible reactions, for example, awful breath, looseness of the bowels and cerebral pains.

It is not necessarily the case that all business diet projects are dangerous. Many depend on sound medicinal and logical standards and can function admirably in certain individuals.

Pick a mindful eating routine program that: instructs you about issues, for example, parcel size, making changes to long haul conduct and smart dieting isn't excessively prohibitive as far as the kind of nourishment you can eat depends on accomplishing steady reasonable weight reduction rather transient fast weight reduction, which is probably not going to last

VERY LOW CALORIE DIET

A very low calorie diet (VLCD) is an eating regimen that includes expending not exactly containing under 3350 kilojoules (800 calories) every day.

While a VLCD can be a successful technique for shedding pounds for some fat individuals, is it not a reasonable or safe strategy for everybody. It would typically possibly be suggested if quick weight reduction was required to diminish the danger of a corpulence related confusion, for example, coronary illness, or on the off chance that you have neglected to shed pounds in spite of ordinary treatment. You should just ever embrace a VLCD under the supervision of an appropriately qualified wellbeing proficient.

OBESITY AND EXERCISE

In the event that you are large and need to lose some weight, it's critical to join good dieting with customary exercise and physical action.

Large people are prescribed to get in any event 2 ½ to 5 hours of moderate-power physical action every week. Moderate force physical movement is any action that expands your heart and breathing rate and may make you sweat, yet you are still ready to hold a typical discussion.

You don't have to do the activity across the board go, you can split it up for the duration of the day into a few separate 15 brief sessions. This degree of movement is a decent begin to help improve your wellbeing and help anticipate advancement of ceaseless conditions, for example, coronary illness and diabetes.

On the off chance that you need to get in shape you may need to develop to 45–an hour of moderate-power physical movement on most days of the week.

Pick exercises that you appreciate, as you are bound to keep doing them. Instances of moderate power physical movement include:

quick strolling

running

swimming

tennis

utilizing a stage coach or comparative at exercise center

Just as moderate force physical action likewise attempt to incorporate quality or obstruction preparing exercise (practicing with loads) on in any event 2 days every week, as this can assist you with consuming fat and increment muscle.

Showing improvement over doing none. In case you're not doing any physical movement right now, intend to begin bit by bit with brief times of activity at once, at that point expand on it to arrive at the prescribed sum.

In the event that you are new to practice or have prior ailments it's a smart thought to converse with your primary care physician before beginning an activity program. Your PCP, physiotherapist or exercise physiologist will have the option to give an activity plan fit to your conditions.

www.ingramcontent.com/pod-product-compliance
Lightning Source LLC
Chambersburg PA
CBHW030535220526
45463CB00007B/2842